£5.00   616.025

FIRST AID  KT-431-759

 St. John Ambulance
Caring for Life

 St. Andrew's Ambulance
Association

LONDON, NEW YORK, MUNICH, MELBOURNE, DELHI

First edition published in Great Britain in 2002
This revised edition published in 2006 by
Dorling Kindersley Limited, 80 Strand, London WC2R 0RL

A Penguin Company

2 4 6 8 10 9 7 5 3 1

Illustration copyright © 2002, 2006 by Dorling Kindersley Limited
Text copyright © 2002, 2006 by St. John Ambulance;
St. Andrew's Ambulance Association; The British Red Cross Society

A CIP catalogue record for this book is available from
the British Library

ISBN 13: 978-1-4053-1573-9
ISBN 10: 1-4053-1573-3

Reproduced in Singapore by Colourscan
Printed and bound in Slovakia by TBB

For further information about the manual
and for on-line updates visit

www.dk.com/firstaidmanual

Discover more at

www.dk.com

St. John Ambulance

St. John Ambulance is England, Wales, and Northern Ireland's leading First Aid charity. Each year, we train over half a million people. We believe that everyone who needs it should receive First Aid, and that no-one should suffer for the lack of trained First Aiders.
• We provide emergency care during local and national sports and cultural events and civil emergencies.
• We encourage personal development for people of all ages.
Visit www.sja.org.uk or call 08700 10 49 50 to get involved.

St. Andrew's Ambulance Association

St. Andrew's Ambulance Association is Scotland's dedicated First Aid charity and provider of First Aid training, services and supplies.
• Our volunteers provide essential First Aid services in communities across Scotland, including cover for events large and small and teaching life-saving skills to others.
• We also supply a full range of First Aid products and training materials to First Aid professionals, industry and the general public.
Visit www.firstaid.org.uk or call 0141 332 4031
St. Andrew's First Aid - Keeping Scotland Safe

British Red Cross

The British Red Cross helps people in crisis, whoever and wherever they are. We are part of a global network of volunteers, responding to natural disasters, conflicts and individual emergencies. The Red Cross is also the world's leading first aid training provider helping people prepare for and respond to accidents and emergencies.
Visit www.redcross.org.uk/firstaid, or call 0870 170 9222

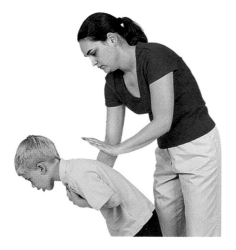

Contents

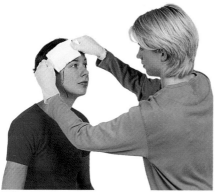

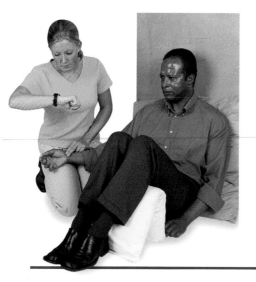

ACTION IN AN EMERGENCY

The main sequence here is for adult casualties. If the casualty is an infant or a child, assess response and breathing then treat as necessary, see special case box.

1 ASSESS SITUATION
- Are there any risks to you or the casualty?

[YES] →
- Put your safety first. If possible, remove the danger from the casualty or, if this is not possible, remove the casualty from danger.
- If it is unsafe, call for emergency help and wait for it to arrive.

[NO] ↓

2 CHECK CASUALTY
- Is the casualty visibly conscious?

[YES] →
- Check for other conditions (opposite) and treat as necessary.
- Summon help if needed.

[NO] ↓

3 CHECK RESPONSE
- Does the casualty respond to your voice or to gentle stimulation?

[YES] →
- Check for other conditions (opposite) and treat as necessary.
- Summon help if needed.

[NO] ↓

4 OPEN AIRWAY; CHECK BREATHING
- Open the casualty's airway and check for breathing (see p.6).
- Is the casualty breathing normally?

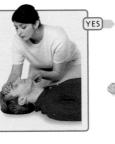

[YES] →
- Place the casualty in the recovery position (see p.9).

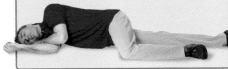

[NO] ↓

ARE YOU ALONE?

[YES] →
- Is the unconsciousness due to drowning?

[NO] ↓

- Ask a helper to call an ambulance and to pass on details of the casualty's condition.
  - ▶ Move on to STEP 5

[YES] ↓
Give five rescue breaths then carry out resuscitation for 1 minute before calling an ambulance.
- ▶ Move on to STEP 5

[NO] ↓
Call an ambulance, then continue the resuscitation sequence.
- ▶ Move on to STEP 5

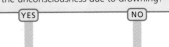

5 COMMENCE CHEST COMPRESSIONS

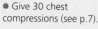

- Give 30 chest compressions (see p.7).

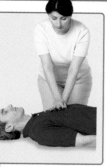

6 COMMENCE RESCUE BREATHS

- Give two rescue breaths (see p.8).

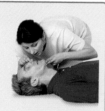

7 CONTINUE CPR

- Continue chest compressions followed by rescue breaths until: emergency help takes over; the casualty starts to breathe normally; or you are too exhausted to continue.

SPECIAL CASE

TREATING CHILDREN AND INFANTS

Assess the child (see p.258 for a child; p.262 for an infant). If not breathing send a helper to call an ambulance.
If you are on your own :

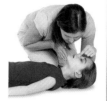

- Give five initial rescue breaths (see p.11 for a child; p.15 for an infant).

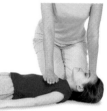

- Give 30 chest compressions (see p.12 for a child; p.15 for an infant), followed by two rescue breaths (CPR).

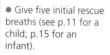

- Continue for 1 minute, then DIAL 999 FOR AN AMBULANCE.
- Continue CPR until: emergency help arrives; the child starts to breathe normally; or you are too exhausted to continue.

TREATMENTS FOR OTHER CONDITIONS

See the following pages for step-by-step treatments:

⚠ WARNING

If at any stage the casualty begins breathing normally, place him in the recovery position (see p.9 for an adult; p.13 for a child; p.14 for an infant).

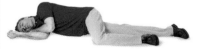

ASSESS THE CASUALTY

1 CHECK RESPONSE

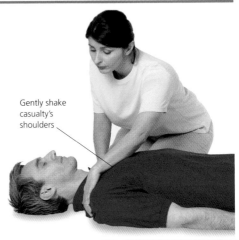

● Ask a question, such as "What's happened?", or give a command, such as "Open your eyes". Speak loudly and clearly.

● Gently shake the casualty's shoulders.

● If there is a response, leave the casualty in the position found and summon help, if needed. Treat any condition found.

● If there is no response, shout for help, then proceed to step 2.

Gently shake casualty's shoulders

2 OPEN AIRWAY

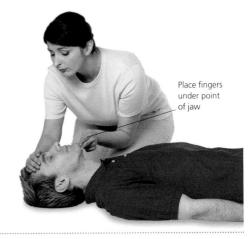

● Place one hand on the casualty's forehead, and gently tilt his head back.

● Place the fingertips of your other hand under the point of the casualty's chin. Lift the chin.

Place fingers under point of jaw

3 CHECK BREATHING

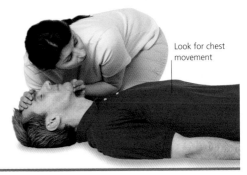

● Look for chest movement, listen for sounds of normal breathing, and feel for breath on your cheek for no more than 10 seconds.

● If the casualty is not breathing, or has agonal breathing, send a helper to DIAL 999 FOR AN AMBULANCE. Begin chest compressions (opposite).

● If he is breathing normally, check for life-threatening conditions such as severe bleeding. Place in recovery position (p.9).

Look for chest movement

CHEST COMPRESSIONS

1 POSITION HANDS FOR CHEST COMPRESSIONS

- Place one hand on the centre of the casualty's chest. This is the point at which you will apply pressure.

- Place the heel of your other hand on top of the first hand, and interlock your fingers. Keep your fingers off the casualty's ribs.

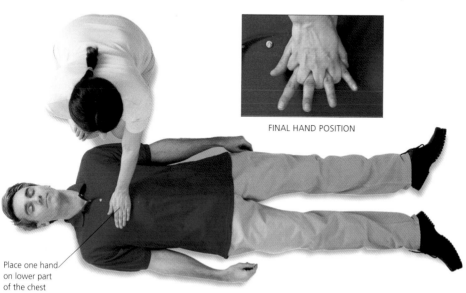

FINAL HAND POSITION

Place one hand on lower part of the chest

2 BEGIN CHEST COMPRESSIONS

- Lean over the casualty, with your arms straight. Press down vertically on the chest, and depress by about 4–5 cm (1½–2 in). Release pressure and let chest recoil.

- Compress the chest 30 times, at a rate of 100 compressions per minute.

- Tilt the head, lift the chin, and give two rescue breaths (p.8).

- Alternate 30 chest compressions with two rescue breaths (CPR).

- Continue CPR until: emergency help arrives and takes over; the casualty starts breathing normally; or you are too exhausted to continue.

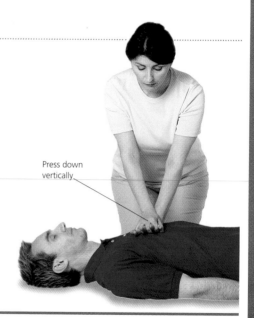

Press down vertically

GIVE RESCUE BREATHS

1 MAKE SURE THAT AIRWAY IS STILL OPEN

● Make sure that the casualty's head remains tilted, by keeping one hand on his forehead and two fingers of the other hand under the tip of his chin.

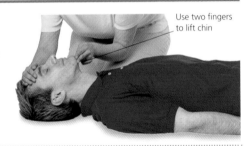

Use two fingers to lift chin

2 PINCH NOSE AND OPEN MOUTH

● Use your thumb and index finger to pinch the soft part of the casualty's nose firmly.

● Make sure that his nostrils are closed to prevent air from escaping.

● Open his mouth.

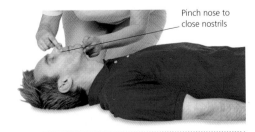

Pinch nose to close nostrils

3 BEGIN RESCUE BREATHS

● Take a breath and place your lips around the casualty's lips, making sure that you form a good seal.

● Blow steadily into the mouth until the chest rises. This should take 1 second. Maintaining head tilt and chin lift, take your mouth away and watch the chest fall. If the chest rises visibly and falls fully, you have given a breath.

● Give two rescue breaths.

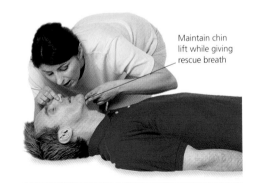

Maintain chin lift while giving rescue breath

4 CONTINUE CHEST COMPRESSIONS AND RESCUE BREATHS

● Repeat 30 chest compressions, followed by two rescue breaths. Continue until: emergency help arrives; the casualty starts breathing normally; or you are too exhausted to continue.

● If the casualty starts breathing normally but remains unconscious, place him in the recovery position (opposite).

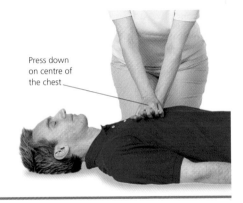

Press down on centre of the chest

RECOVERY POSITION

1 POSITION ARM AND STRAIGHTEN LEGS

- Kneel beside the casualty.

- Remove spectacles and any bulky objects (such as mobile phones or large bunches of keys) from the pockets. Straighten his legs.

- Place the arm nearest to you at right angles to the casualty's body, with the elbow bent and the palm facing upwards.

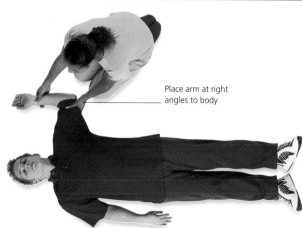

Place arm at right angles to body

2 POSITION FAR ARM, HAND, AND KNEE

- Bring the arm farthest from you across the casualty's chest and hold the back of his hand against the cheek nearest to you.

- Using your other hand, grasp the far leg just above the knee and pull it up until the foot is flat on the floor.

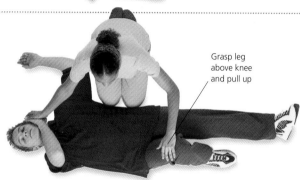

Grasp leg above knee and pull up

3 ROLL CASUALTY TOWARDS YOU

- Keeping the casualty's hand pressed against his cheek, pull on the far leg and roll him towards you and on to his side.

- Adjust the upper leg so that both the hip and knee are bent at right angles.

- Tilt the head back to ensure that the airway remains open.

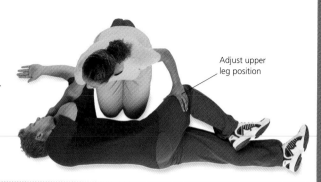

Adjust upper leg position

4 DIAL 999 FOR AN AMBULANCE, IF NOT ALREADY DONE

- Ideally, ask a helper to make the call while you wait with the casualty.

- Monitor and record vital signs – level of response, pulse, and breathing.

ASSESS THE CHILD

1 CHECK RESPONSE

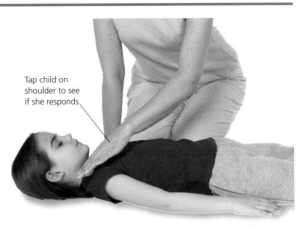

Tap child on shoulder to see if she responds

- Ask the child a question, such as "Can you hear me?". Speak loudly and clearly.

- Gently tap her on the shoulder.

- If there is a response, leave the child in the position found and summon help, if needed. Treat any condition found.

- If there is no response, then proceed to step 2.

2 OPEN AIRWAY

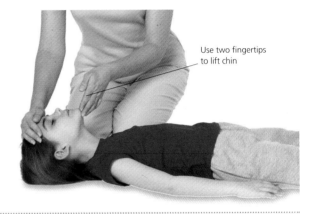

Use two fingertips to lift chin

- Place one hand on the child's forehead. Gently tilt the head back.

- Place the fingertips of your other hand under the point of the child's chin. Lift the chin.

3 CHECK BREATHING

- Look for chest movement, listen for sounds of breathing, and feel for breath on your cheek. Do this for no more than 10 seconds.

- If the child is not breathing, send a helper to
DIAL 999 FOR AN AMBULANCE. Begin rescue breathing (opposite).

- If breathing normally, check for life-threatening conditions such as severe bleeding. Place in the recovery position (p.13).

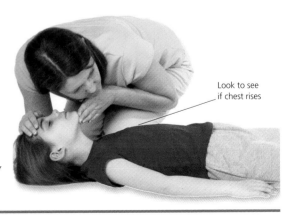

Look to see if chest rises

GIVE RESCUE BREATHS

1 MAKE SURE THAT AIRWAY IS STILL OPEN

● Make sure that the child's head remains tilted, by keeping one hand on her forehead and two fingers of the other hand on the point of her chin.

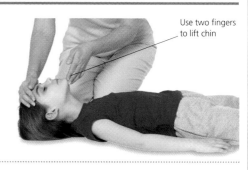

Use two fingers to lift chin

2 CLEAR HER AIRWAY

● Using your fingertips, pick out any visible obstructions from the child's mouth. Do not do a finger sweep.

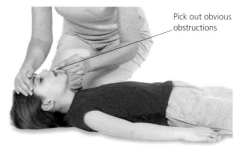

Pick out obvious obstructions

3 PINCH NOSE AND OPEN MOUTH

● Use your thumb and index finger to pinch the soft part of the child's nose firmly. Make sure that her nostrils are closed to prevent air from escaping.

● Open the child's mouth.

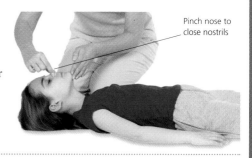

Pinch nose to close nostrils

4 GIVE RESCUE BREATHS

● Take a breath and place your lips around the child's lips, making sure that you form an airtight seal.

● Blow steadily into the mouth for 1 second; the chest should rise. Maintaining head tilt and chin lift, take your mouth away and watch the chest fall. If the chest rises visibly and falls fully, you have given a breath.

● Give five rescue breaths.

● Begin chest compressions (p.12).

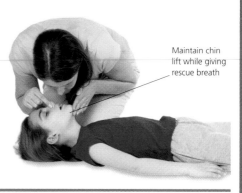

Maintain chin lift while giving rescue breath

CHEST COMPRESSIONS

1 POSITION HANDS FOR CHEST COMPRESSIONS

● Place the heel of one hand on the centre of the child's chest. This is the point at which you will apply pressure.

● Use the heel of only one hand to apply pressure. Lift your fingers to ensure that you do not apply pressure to the child's ribs.

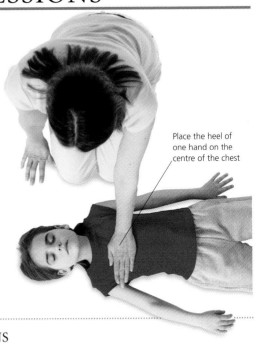

Place the heel of one hand on the centre of the chest

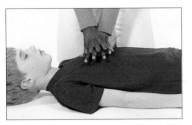

FOR LARGER CHILD OR SMALL RESCUER, USE TWO HANDS FOR CHEST COMPRESSIONS

2 BEGIN CHEST COMPRESSIONS AND RESCUE BREATHS

● Lean well over the child, with your arm straight. Press down vertically on the breastbone, and depress the chest by one-third of its depth. Release the pressure and allow the chest to come back up.

● Compress the chest 30 times, at a rate of 100 compressions per minute.

● Give two rescue breaths (p.11).

● Continue to alternate 30 chest compressions with two rescue breaths for 1 minute. Then if you are alone, DIAL 999 FOR AN AMBULANCE

● Continue CPR until: emergency help takes over; the child starts to breathe normally; or you are too exhausted to continue.

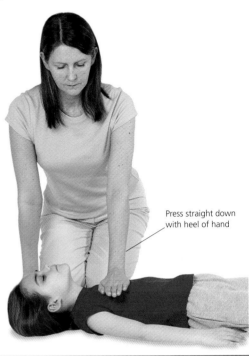

Press straight down with heel of hand

RECOVERY POSITION

1 POSITION ARM AND STRAIGHTEN LEGS

- Kneel beside the casualty.

- Remove spectacles and any bulky objects from the pockets.

- Straighten her legs.

- Place the arm nearest to you at right angles to the child's body, with the elbow bent and the palm facing upwards.

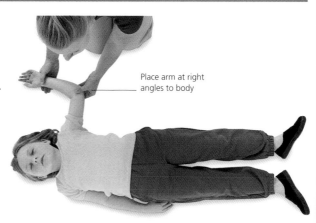

Place arm at right angles to body

2 POSITION FAR ARM, HAND, AND KNEE

- Bring the arm farthest from you across the child's chest.

- Hold the back of her hand against the cheek nearest to you.

- Using your other hand, grasp the far leg just above the knee and pull it up until the foot is flat on the floor.

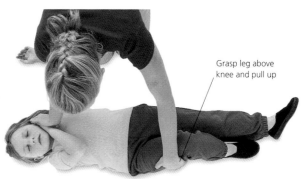

Grasp leg above knee and pull up

3 ROLL CHILD TOWARDS YOU

- Keeping the child's hand pressed against her cheek, pull on the far leg and roll her towards you and on to her side.

- Adjust the child's upper leg so that both the hip and the knee are bent at right angles.

- Tilt her head back to ensure that the airway remains open.

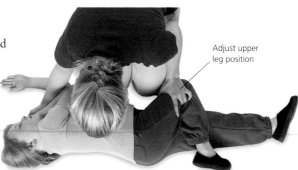

Adjust upper leg position

4 DIAL 999 FOR AN AMBULANCE, IF NOT ALREADY DONE

- Monitor and record vital signs – level of response, pulse, and breathing.

ASSESS THE INFANT

1 CHECK RESPONSE

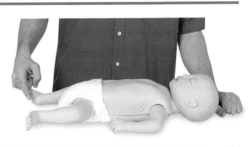

- Gently tap or flick the sole of the infant's foot. Never shake an infant.

- If there is a response, take the baby with you to summon help if needed.

- If no response, shout for help; go to step 2.

2 OPEN AIRWAY

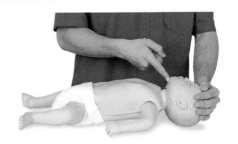

- Place one hand on the infant's forehead, and very gently tilt the head back.

- Then place one fingertip of your other hand under the point of the infant's chin. Lift the chin.

3 CHECK BREATHING

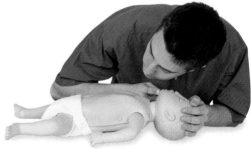

- Look for chest movement, listen for sounds of normal breathing, and feel for breath on your cheek for no more than 10 seconds.

- If the infant is not breathing, send a helper to **DIAL 999 FOR AN AMBULANCE** Begin rescue breathing (opposite).

- If breathing normally, check for injuries and hold in the recovery position (below).

RECOVERY POSITION

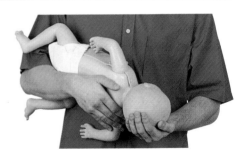

- Cradle the infant in your arms, with his head tilted downwards to prevent him from choking on his tongue or inhaling vomit.

- Monitor and record vital signs – level of response, pulse, and breathing – until medical help arrives.

GIVE RESCUE BREATHS

1 MAKE SURE AIRWAY IS OPEN AND CLEAR

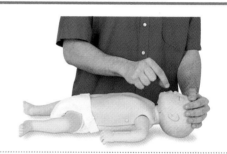

● Make sure that the airway remains open, by keeping the infant's head tilted back and the chin lifted.

● Using your fingertips, pick out any visible obstructions. Do not do a finger sweep.

2 GIVE RESCUE BREATHS

● Take a breath and place your lips around the infant's mouth and nose, making sure that you form an airtight seal.

● Blow steadily into the mouth for 1 second; the chest should rise. Maintaining head tilt and chin lift, take your mouth away and watch the chest fall. If the chest rises visibly and falls fully, you have given a breath.

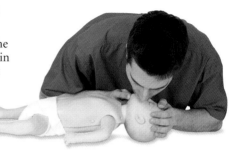

● Give five rescue breaths.

● Begin chest compressions (below).

CHEST COMPRESSIONS

1 POSITION FINGERS FOR CHEST COMPRESSIONS

● Place the tips of your index and middle fingers on the centre of the infant's chest.

Place fingertips on centre of chest

2 GIVE CHEST COMPRESSIONS AND RESCUE BREATHS

● Press down vertically, depressing chest by one-third of its depth. Release pressure and let chest recoil. Give 30 compressions at 100 per minute.

● Give two rescue breaths. Alternate 30 chest compressions with two rescue breaths. Continue CPR until emergency help takes over; the infant starts breathing normally; or you are too exhausted to continue.

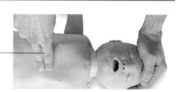
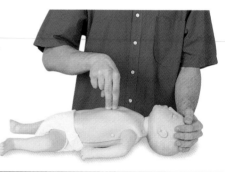

CHOKING ADULT

RECOGNITION

Ask casualty "Are you choking?"

Mild obstruction
- Difficulty in speaking, coughing and breathing.

Severe obstruction
- Inability to speak, cough, or breathe.
- Eventual loss of consciousness.

PRECAUTIONS
- If the casualty loses consciousness, open airway and check breathing. Be ready to give chest compressions and rescue breaths (pp.7–8).
- Do not do a finger sweep of the mouth.

ACTION

GIVE UP TO FIVE
BACK BLOWS
CHECK MOUTH

GIVE UP TO FIVE
ABDOMINAL
THRUSTS
CHECK MOUTH

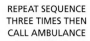

REPEAT SEQUENCE
THREE TIMES THEN
CALL AMBULANCE

REPEAT SEQUENCE
UNTIL HELP ARRIVES
OR CASUALTY IS
UNCONSCIOUS

1 GIVE UP TO FIVE BACK BLOWS
- Encourage the casualty to cough to try to remove the obstruction.
- If the casualty cannot speak, cough, or breathe, bend him forwards.
- Give up to five sharp blows between the shoulder blades with the heel of your hand. Check his mouth.
- If choking persists, proceed to step 2.

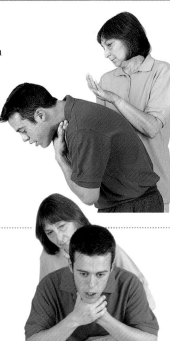

2 HOLD CASUALTY FROM BEHIND
- Stand behind the casualty.
- Put both arms around him, and put one fist between his navel and the bottom of his breastbone.

3 GIVE UP TO FIVE ABDOMINAL THRUSTS
- Grasp your fist with your other hand, and pull sharply inwards and upwards up to five times.
- If the obstruction is still not cleared, recheck the mouth for any object and remove it if possible.

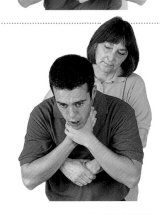

4 REPEAT ENTIRE SEQUENCE
- Repeat steps 1–3 until the obstruction clears. If after three cycles it still has not cleared, DIAL 999 FOR AN AMBULANCE
- Continue the sequence until help arrives; the obstruction is cleared; or the casualty becomes unconscious (see PRECAUTIONS, left).

CHOKING CHILD (1 year to puberty)

RECOGNITION

Ask child "Are you choking ?"

Mild obstruction

- Difficulty in speaking coughing, and breathing.

Severe obstruction

- Inability to speak, cough, or breathe.
- Eventual loss of consciousness.

PRECAUTIONS

- If the child loses consciousness, open airway and check breathing. Be ready to give rescue breaths and chest compressions (pp.11–12).
- Do not do a finger sweep of the mouth.

ACTION

GIVE UP TO FIVE
BACK BLOWS
CHECK MOUTH

GIVE UP TO FIVE
ABDOMINAL
THRUSTS
CHECK MOUTH

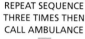

REPEAT SEQUENCE
THREE TIMES THEN
CALL AMBULANCE

REPEAT SEQUENCE
UNTIL HELP ARRIVES
OR CHILD IS
UNCONSCIOUS

1 GIVE UP TO FIVE BACK BLOWS

- Encourage the child to cough.
- If the child is unable to speak, cough, or breathe, bend him forwards.
- Give up to five sharp blows between his shoulder blades using the heel of your hand. Check his mouth.
- If choking persists, proceed to step 2.

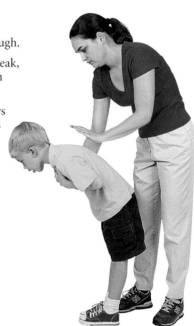

2 GIVE UP TO FIVE ABDOMINAL THRUSTS

- Stand behind the child with both arms around the upper abdomen. Make a fist, and place it between the child's navel and the bottom of his breastbone.
- Grasp your fist with your hand. Pull sharply inwards and upwards up to five times. Check the child's mouth.
- If choking persists, proceed to step 3.

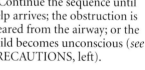

3 REPEAT ENTIRE SEQUENCE

- Repeat steps 1 and 2 until the obstruction clears.
- If after three cycles the obstruction still has not cleared, DIAL 999 FOR AN AMBULANCE

- Continue the sequence until help arrives; the obstruction is cleared from the airway; or the child becomes unconscious (*see* PRECAUTIONS, left).

CHOKING INFANT (under 1 year)

RECOGNITION

Mild obstruction
- Able to cough but difficulty making any noise or breathing.

Severe obstruction
- Inability to cough or make any noise, eventual unconsciousness.

PRECAUTIONS

- If the infant loses consciousness, give rescue breaths and chest compressions (p.15).
- Do not do a finger sweep of the mouth.
- Do not use abdominal thrusts.

ACTION

GIVE UP TO FIVE
BACK BLOWS
CHECK MOUTH

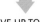

GIVE UP TO FIVE
CHEST THRUSTS
CHECK MOUTH

REPEAT SEQUENCE
THREE TIMES THEN
CALL AMBULANCE

REPEAT
SEQUENCE UNTIL
HELP ARRIVES OR
INFANT IS
UNCONSCIOUS

1 GIVE UP TO FIVE BACK BLOWS

- If the infant cannot cough or breathe, lay him face down along your forearm, with head low, and supporting his body and head.
- Give up to five back blows between the shoulder blades with the heel of your hand.
- If choking persists, proceed to step 2.

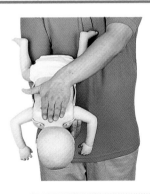

2 CHECK INFANT'S MOUTH

- Turn the infant face up along your other forearm.
- Use your fingertips to pick out any visible obstructions.
- If choking persists, proceed to step 3.

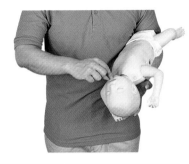

3 GIVE UP TO FIVE CHEST THRUSTS

- Place two fingertips on the lower half of the infant's breastbone, one finger's breadth below the nipples.
- Give up to five sharp thrusts inwards and towards the head at rate of one every 3 seconds.
- Check the mouth again.
- If choking persists, proceed to step 4.

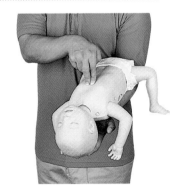

4 REPEAT ENTIRE SEQUENCE

- Repeat steps 1–3 three times.
- If the obstruction still does not clear, take the infant with you to **DIAL 999 FOR AN AMBULANCE**
- Continue the sequence until help arrives; the obstruction is cleared from the airway; or the infant becomes unconscious (*see* PRECAUTIONS, left).

ASTHMA ATTACK

RECOGNITION

- Difficulty in breathing.

There may be:
- Wheezing.
- Difficulty in speaking.
- Grey–blue skin.
- Exhaustion and possible loss of consciousness.

PRECAUTIONS

- Do not lay the casualty down.
- Do not use a preventer inhaler.
- If the attack is severe, or if the inhaler has no effect after 5 minutes, or if the casualty is getting worse
DIAL 999 FOR AN AMBULANCE
- If the casualty loses consciousness, open the airway and check breathing (p.6). Be prepared to give chest compressions and rescue breaths if needed.

ACTION

ALLOW CASUALTY
TO USE RELIEVER
INHALER

MAKE CASUALTY
COMFORTABLE

ENCOURAGE
CASUALTY TO
BREATHE SLOWLY

1 MAKE CASUALTY COMFORTABLE

- Keep calm and reassure the casualty.

- Help her into the position that she finds most comfortable; sitting slightly forwards and supporting the upper body by leaning the arms on a firm surface is usually best.

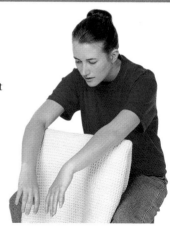

2 ALLOW CASUALTY TO USE RELIEVER INHALER

- Help the casualty to find her reliever inhaler (it is usually blue).

- Encourage the casualty to use the inhaler; it should take effect within minutes.

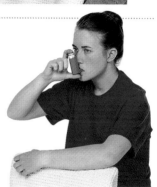

3 ENCOURAGE CASUALTY TO BREATHE SLOWLY

- If the attack does not ease within 3 minutes, encourage the casualty to take another dose from her inhaler and to breathe slowly and deeply.

- Tell the casualty to inform her doctor of the attack if it is severe or if it is her first attack.

- If the attack is severe, if the inhaler has no effect after 5 minutes, or if the casualty is getting worse, **DIAL 999 FOR AN AMBULANCE**

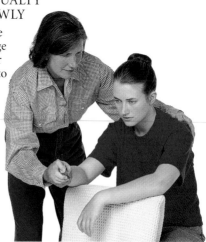

SHOCK

RECOGNITION

- Rapid pulse.
- Pale, cold, clammy skin.
- Sweating.

Later:
- Grey–blue skin, especially inside lips.
- Weakness and giddiness.
- Nausea or thirst.
- Rapid, shallow breathing.
- Weak pulse.

Eventually:
- Restlessness.
- Gasping for air.
- Unconsciousness.

PRECAUTIONS

- Do not leave the casualty unattended, except to call an ambulance.
- Do not let the casualty smoke, eat, drink, or move.

ACTION

HELP CASUALTY
TO LIE DOWN

LOOSEN TIGHT
CLOTHING

CALL AMBULANCE

MONITOR
CASUALTY

1 HELP CASUALTY TO LIE DOWN

- Use a blanket to insulate the casualty from the ground.
- Raise and support her legs as high as possible.
- Treat any cause of shock, such as bleeding.

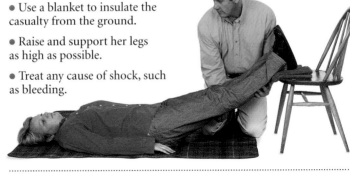

2 LOOSEN TIGHT CLOTHING

- Undo anything that constricts her neck, chest and waist.
- Cover her with a blanket.

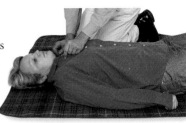

3 DIAL 999 FOR AN AMBULANCE

- If possible, send a helper to call an ambulance.
- The caller should give the controller details about the cause of shock, if known.

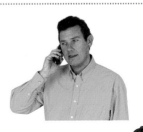

4 MONITOR BREATHING, PULSE, AND RESPONSE

- Monitor and record vital signs – level of response, pulse, and breathing.
- If the casualty becomes unconscious, open the airway and check breathing (p.6). Be ready to give chest compressions and rescue breaths.

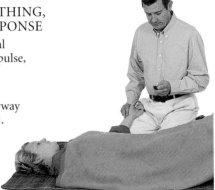

ANAPHYLACTIC SHOCK

RECOGNITION

- Anxiety.
- Red, blotchy skin.
- Swelling of tongue and throat.
- Puffiness around eyes.
- Impaired breathing, possibly with wheezing and gasping for air.
- Signs of shock.

PRECAUTIONS

- Check to see if the casualty is carrying an auto-injector or a syringe of epinephrine (adrenaline). If necessary, assist the casualty to use it. It can save his life when given promptly.
- If the casualty loses consciousness, open the airway and check breathing (p.6). If breathing, place him in the recovery position. Be prepared to give chest compressions and rescue breaths if necessary.

ACTION

CALL
AMBULANCE

⬇

HELP TO RELIEVE
SYMPTOMS

⬇

MONITOR
CASUALTY

1 DIAL 999 FOR AN AMBULANCE

- Pass on as much information as possible about the cause of the allergy.

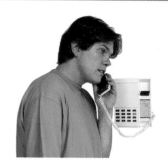

2 HELP TO RELIEVE SYMPTOMS

- Check whether the casualty is carrying a syringe or an auto-injector of epinephrine (adrenaline). Help the casualty to find and use it if necessary.

- Help the casualty to sit in a position that eases any breathing difficulties.

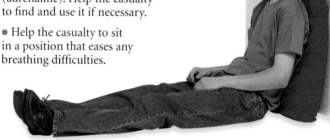

3 MONITOR CASUALTY

- Monitor and record vital signs – level of response, pulse, and breathing – until help arrives.

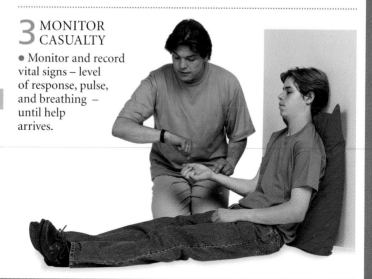

SEVERE BLEEDING

PRECAUTIONS

- Do not apply a tourniquet.
- If there is an embedded object in the wound, apply pressure on either side of the wound, and pad around it before bandaging.
- Wear gloves, if available, to protect against infection.
- If the casualty loses consciousness, open the airway and check breathing (p.6). If she is breathing, place her in the recovery position. Be ready to give chest compressions and rescue breaths if needed.

1 APPLY PRESSURE TO WOUND

- Put on gloves if available. Remove or cut any clothing over the wound.
- Place a sterile dressing or non-fluffy pad over the wound. Apply firm pressure with your fingers or the palm of your hand.

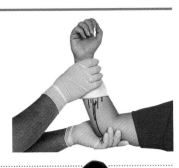

2 RAISE AND SUPPORT INJURED PART

- Raise the injured part above the level of the casualty's heart.
- Handle the injured part gently if you suspect that the injury involves a fracture.
- Help the casualty to lie down.

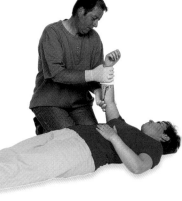

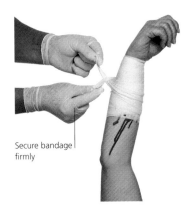

ACTION

APPLY PRESSURE TO WOUND

RAISE AND SUPPORT INJURED PART

BANDAGE WOUND

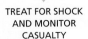

CALL AMBULANCE

TREAT FOR SHOCK AND MONITOR CASUALTY

3 BANDAGE WOUND

- Apply a sterile dressing over the pad, and bandage firmly in place.
- Bandage another pad on top if blood seeps through. If blood seeps through the second pad, remove all dressings and apply a fresh one, ensuring that it exerts pressure on the bleeding area.
- Check the circulation beyond the bandages at intervals; loosen them if necessary.

Secure bandage firmly

4 DIAL 999 FOR AN AMBULANCE

- Give details of the site of the injury and the extent of the bleeding when you telephone.

5 TREAT FOR SHOCK; MONITOR CASUALTY

- Treat for shock (p.20). Monitor and record vital signs – level of response, pulse, and breathing.

HEART ATTACK

RECOGNITION

There may be:
- Vice-like chest pain, spreading to one or both arms.
- Breathlessness.
- Discomfort, like indigestion, in upper abdomen.
- Sudden faintness.
- Sudden collapse.
- Sense of impending doom.
- Ashen skin and blueness at lips.
- Rapid, then weakening, pulse.
- Profuse sweating.

PRECAUTIONS

- Do not give fluids.
- If the casualty loses consciousness, open the airway and check breathing (p.6). If the casualty is not breathing normally, or has agonal breathing, be ready to give chest compressions.

ACTION

MAKE CASUALTY COMFORTABLE

↓

CALL AMBULANCE

↓

GIVE CASUALTY ASPIRIN

↓

MONITOR CASUALTY

1 MAKE CASUALTY COMFORTABLE

- Help the casualty into a half-sitting position.
- Support his head, shoulders, and knees.
- Reassure the casualty.

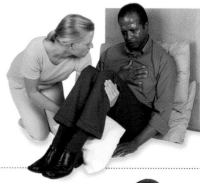

2 DIAL 999 FOR AN AMBULANCE

- Tell the controller that you suspect a heart attack.
- Call the casualty's doctor as well, if he asks you to do so.

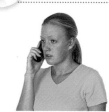

3 GIVE CASUALTY MEDICATION

- If the casualty is conscious, give one tablet of aspirin to be *chewed* slowly.
- If the casualty is carrying tablets or a puffer aerosol for angina, allow him to administer it himself. Help him if necessary.

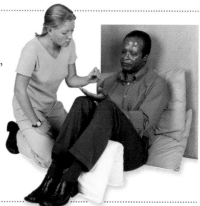

4 MONITOR CASUALTY

- Encourage the casualty to rest. Keep any bystanders at a distance.
- Monitor and record vital signs – level of response, pulse, and breathing – until help arrives.

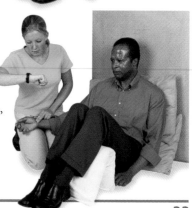

HEAD INJURY

RECOGNITION

There may be:
- Head wound.
- Impaired consciousness.

PRECAUTIONS

- Wear gloves, if available, to protect against infection.
- If the casualty loses consciousness, open the airway and check breathing (p.6). If she is breathing, place her in the recovery position. Be ready to give chest compressions and rescue breaths if needed.
- If the bleeding does not stop, reapply pressure and add a second pad.
- Always suspect the possibility of a neck (spinal) injury (opposite).

ACTION

CONTROL BLEEDING

⬇

SECURE DRESSING WITH BANDAGE

⬇

HELP CASUALTY TO LIE DOWN

⬇

CALL AMBULANCE

1 CONTROL BLEEDING

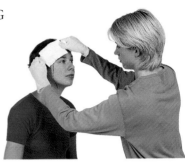

- Put on disposable gloves if available.
- Replace any displaced skin flaps over the wound.
- Place a sterile dressing or a clean, non-fluffy pad over the wound and apply firm, direct pressure with your hand.

2 SECURE DRESSING WITH BANDAGE

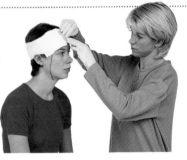

- Secure the dressing over the wound with a roller bandage.

3 HELP CASUALTY TO LIE DOWN

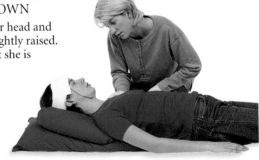

- Ensure that her head and shoulders are slightly raised.
- Make sure that she is comfortable.

4 DIAL 999 FOR AN AMBULANCE

- Monitor and record vital signs – level of response, pulse, and breathing – until help arrives.

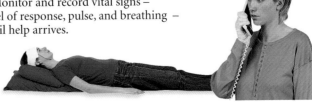

SPINAL INJURY

RECOGNITION

- Pain in neck or back.
- A step or twist in the curve of the spine.
- Tenderness over the spine.

There may be:
- Weakness or loss of movement in limbs.
- Loss of sensation, or abnormal sensation.
- Loss of bladder and/or bowel control.
- Difficulty breathing.

PRECAUTIONS

- Do not move the casualty unless she is in danger.
- If the casualty loses consciousness, open the airway by gently lifting the jaw but not tilting the head; check breathing (p.6). Place her in the recovery position only if the airway cannot be maintained. Be ready to give chest compressions and rescue breaths if needed.

ACTION

STEADY AND
SUPPORT HEAD

CALL AMBULANCE

1 STEADY AND SUPPORT HEAD

- Reassure the casualty and tell her not to move.
- Keep the head, neck, and spine aligned by placing your hands on the sides of the head to hold the head still.

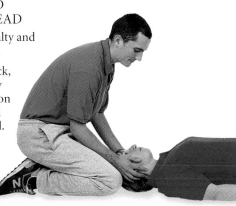

2 SUPPORT CASUALTY'S NECK

- Ask a helper to place rolled towels or other padding around the casualty's neck and shoulders.
- Keep holding her head throughout, until medical help arrives.

3 DIAL 999 FOR AN AMBULANCE

- If possible, ask a helper to call an ambulance and say that a spinal injury is suspected.
- Monitor and record vital signs – level of response, pulse, and breathing.

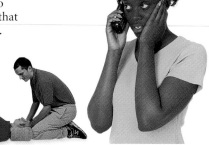

SEIZURES IN ADULTS

RECOGNITION

- Sudden loss of consciousness.
- Rigidity and arching of the back.
- Convulsive movements.
- Muscle relaxation.
- Regaining of consciousness.
- Grey–blue tinge to skin.

PRECAUTIONS

- Do not use force to restrain the casualty.
- If the casualty is unconscious for more than 10 minutes, is having repeated seizures, or it is her first seizure, DIAL 999 FOR AN AMBULANCE Note the time when the seizure starts and the duration of the seizure.

ACTION

PROTECT CASUALTY

PROTECT HEAD AND LOOSEN TIGHT CLOTHING

PLACE CASUALTY IN RECOVERY POSITION

MONITOR CASUALTY

1 PROTECT CASUALTY

- Try to ease her fall.
- Talk to her calmly and reassuringly.
- Clear away any potentially dangerous objects to prevent injury to the casualty.
- Ask bystanders to keep clear.

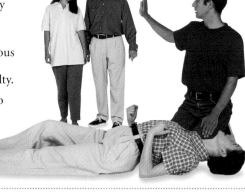

2 PROTECT HEAD AND LOOSEN TIGHT CLOTHING

- If possible, cushion the casualty's head with soft material until the seizures cease.
- Undo any tight clothing around the casualty's neck.

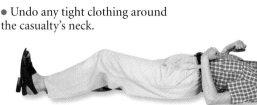

3 PLACE CASUALTY IN RECOVERY POSITION

- Once the seizures have stopped, open the airway and check breathing (p.6); then place the casualty in the recovery position (p.9).
- Monitor and record vital signs – level of response, pulse, and breathing.

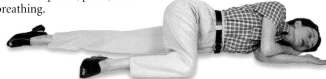

SEIZURES IN CHILDREN

RECOGNITION

- Violent muscle twitching, clenched fists, and arched back.

There may be:
- Fever.
- Twitching of the face.
- Breath-holding.
- Drooling at the mouth.
- Loss of, or impaired, consciousness.

PRECAUTIONS

- Do not let the child become chilled.
- If the child loses consciousness, open the airway and check breathing (p.10, p.14). Be ready to give rescue breaths and chest compressions if needed (pp.11–12, p.15).

ACTION

PROTECT CHILD FROM INJURY

⬇

COOL CHILD

⬇

SPONGE WITH TEPID WATER

⬇

PUT CHILD IN RECOVERY POSITION

⬇

CALL AMBULANCE; MONITOR CHILD

1 PROTECT CHILD FROM INJURY

- Clear away any nearby objects.
- Surround the child with soft padding.

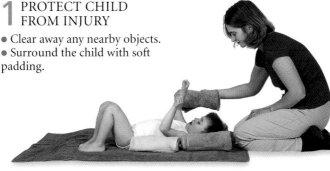

2 COOL CHILD

- Remove his clothing.
- Ensure a good supply of cool air.

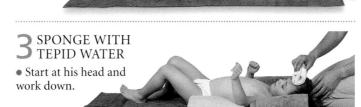

3 SPONGE WITH TEPID WATER

- Start at his head and work down.

4 PUT CHILD IN RECOVERY POSITION

- Once the seizures have stopped, open the airway and check breathing (p.10, p.14), then put the child in the recovery position (p.13, p.14).

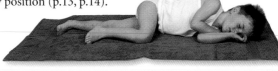

5 DIAL 999 FOR AN AMBULANCE AND MONITOR CHILD

- Monitor and record vital signs – level of response, pulse, and breathing – until help arrives.

BROKEN BONES

RECOGNITION

- Distortion, swelling, and bruising at the injury site.
- Pain and difficulty in moving the injured part.

There may be:

- Bending, twisting, or shortening of a limb.
- A wound, possibly with bone ends protruding.

1 STEADY AND SUPPORT INJURED PART

- Help the casualty to support the affected part, above and below the injury, in the most comfortable position.

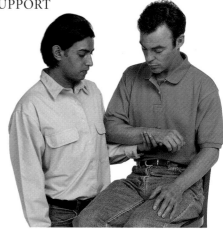

PRECAUTIONS

- Do not attempt to bandage the injury if medical assistance is on its way.
- Do not attempt to move an injured limb unnecessarily.
- Do not allow a casualty with a suspected fracture to eat, drink, or smoke.

2 PROTECT INJURY WITH PADDING

- Place padding, such as towels or cushions, around the affected part, and support it in position.
- If there is an open wound, cover it with a large, sterile dressing or a clean, non-fluffy pad and bandage it in place.

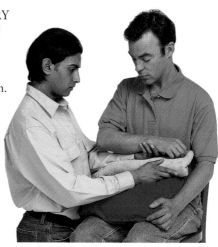

ACTION

STEADY AND SUPPORT INJURED PART

PROTECT INJURY WITH PADDING

TAKE OR SEND CASUALTY TO HOSPITAL

3 TAKE OR SEND CASUALTY TO HOSPITAL

- Call an ambulance if necessary.
- Treat the casualty for shock (p.20).
- Monitor and record vital signs – level of response, pulse, and breathing.

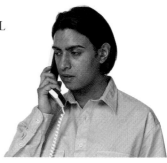

BURNS

RECOGNITION

- Reddened skin.
- Pain in the area of the burn.
- Swelling and blistering of the skin.

PRECAUTIONS

- Do not apply lotions, ointment, or fat to a burn.
- Do not touch the burn or burst any blisters.
- Do not remove anything sticking to the burn.
- If the burn is to the face, do not cover it. Keep cooling with water until help arrives.
- If the burn is caused by chemicals, cool for at least 20 minutes.

ACTION

COOL BURN

REMOVE ANY CONSTRICTIONS

COVER BURN

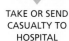

TAKE OR SEND CASUALTY TO HOSPITAL

1 COOL BURN

- Make the casualty comfortable.
- Pour cold liquid on the burn for at least 10 minutes.
- Watch for signs of smoke inhalation, such as difficulty breathing.

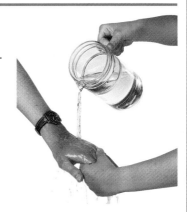

2 REMOVE ANY CONSTRICTIONS

- Put on disposable gloves if available.
- Carefully remove any clothing or jewellery from the area before it starts to swell. However, do not try to remove any clothing that is sticking to the burn.

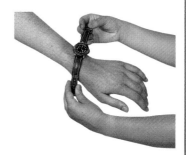

3 COVER BURN

- Cover the burn and the surrounding area with a sterile dressing, clean non-fluffy material, cling film, or a plastic bag.
- Reassure the casualty.

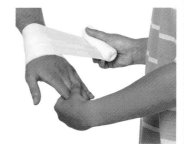

4 TAKE OR SEND CASUALTY TO HOSPITAL

- Call an ambulance if necessary.
- Treat the casualty for shock (p.20).
- Monitor and record vital signs – level of response, pulse, and breathing.

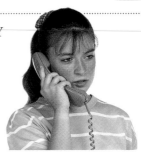

EYE INJURY

RECOGNITION

- Intense pain in the affected eye.
- Spasm of the eyelids.

There may also be:
- A visible wound.
- A bloodshot eye, even if wound is not visible.
- Partial or total loss of vision.
- Leakage of blood or clear fluid from the injured eye.

PRECAUTIONS

- Do not touch the eye or any contact lens in it, and do not allow the casualty to rub the eye.
- Do not try to remove any object embedded in the eye.
- If it will be some time before medical aid is available, bandage an eye pad in place over the injured eye.

ACTION

SUPPORT CASUALTY'S HEAD
⬇
GIVE EYE DRESSING TO CASUALTY
⬇
TAKE OR SEND CASUALTY TO HOSPITAL

1 SUPPORT CASUALTY'S HEAD

- Lay the casualty on her back, holding her head on your knees to keep it as still as possible.
- Tell the casualty to keep her "good" eye still; movement of the uninjured eye will cause the injured one to move as well, which may damage it further.

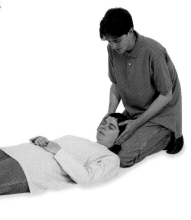

2 GIVE EYE DRESSING TO CASUALTY

- Give the casualty a sterile dressing or clean non-fluffy pad. Ask her to hold it over the injured eye and to keep her uninjured eye closed.
- Hold the casualty's head steady.

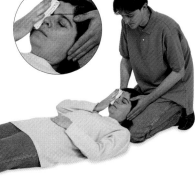

3 TAKE OR SEND CASUALTY TO HOSPITAL

- Ensure that the casualty is transported lying down. Call an ambulance if you cannot transport her in the position in which she was treated.

Provide support for casualty's head

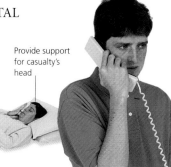

SWALLOWED POISONS

RECOGNITION

- Vomiting that may be bloodstained.
- Impaired consciousness.
- Empty bottles and containers nearby.
- History of ingestion/exposure.
- Pain or burning sensation.

PRECAUTIONS

- Do not attempt to induce vomiting.
- If the casualty loses consciousness, make sure that there is no vomit or other matter in the mouth. Open the airway and check breathing (p.6). Be ready to give chest compressions and rescue breaths if needed.
- When giving rescue breaths, use a face shield or pocket mask for protection if there are chemicals on the casualty's mouth.

ACTION

CHECK WHAT
CASUALTY HAS
SWALLOWED

⬇

CALL AMBULANCE

⬇

MONITOR
CASUALTY

1 CHECK WHAT CASUALTY HAS SWALLOWED

- If the casualty is conscious, ask what she has swallowed and reassure her.

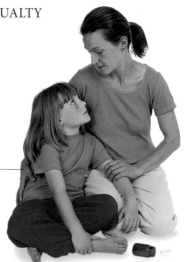

Reassure casualty as you find out what she swallowed

2 DIAL 999 FOR AN AMBULANCE

- Give as much information as possible about the swallowed poison. This information will help doctors to give the casualty the appropriate treatment.

- Monitor and record vital signs – level of response, pulse, and breathing – until help arrives.

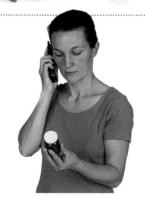

3 IF CASUALTY'S LIPS ARE BURNT

- If the swallowed substance has burnt the casualty's lips, give her frequent sips of cold water or milk.

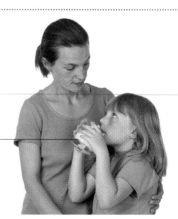

Give casualty cool, soothing drink such as milk

OBSERVATION CHARTS

Fill in the following charts every time you attend to a casualty.
- On the first chart, place a dot opposite the appropriate score at each time interval.
- On the second chart, tick the appropriate pulse and breathing rates at each interval.
- The completed form should stay with the casualty when he leaves your care.

LEVEL OF RESPONSE CHART

DATE..........................CASUALTY'S NAME...

OBSERVATION	RESPONSE/SCORE	Time of observation (minutes)					
		0	10	20	30	40	50
Eyes Observe for reaction while testing other responses.	Open spontaneously 4 Open to speech 3 Open to painful stimulus 2 No response 1						
Speech When testing responses, speak clearly and directly, close to casualty's ear.	Responds sensibly to questions 5 Seems confused 4 Uses inappropriate words 3 Incomprehensible sounds 2 No response 1						
Movement Apply painful stimulus: pinch ear lobe or skin on back of hand.	Obeys commands 6 Points to pain 5 Withdraws from painful stimulus 4 Bends limbs in response to pain 3 Straightens limbs in response to pain 2 No response 1						
	TOTAL SCORE						

PULSE AND BREATHING CHECK CHART

DATE..........................CASUALTY'S NAME...

PULSE/BREATHING	RATE	Time of observation (minutes)					
		0	10	20	30	40	50
Pulse (beats per minute) Take pulse at wrist or at neck on adult, or at inner arm on baby. Note the rate, and whether beats are weak (w) or strong (s), regular (reg) or irregular (irreg).	Over 110						
	101–110						
	91–100						
	81–90						
	71–80						
	61–70						
	Below 61						
Breathing (breaths per minute) Note rate, and whether breathing is quiet (q) or noisy (n), easy (e) or difficult (diff).	Over 40						
	31–40						
	21–30						
	11–20						
	Below 11						

mountains and rivers

" In the new way of things, the community is essential to the creative act; the solitary poet figure and the ' name ' author will become less and less relevant. Hence I prefer to be with my friends — which is the creative context.
We are on top of the live volcano of Suwa-no-se island, at sunrise, chanting mantras."

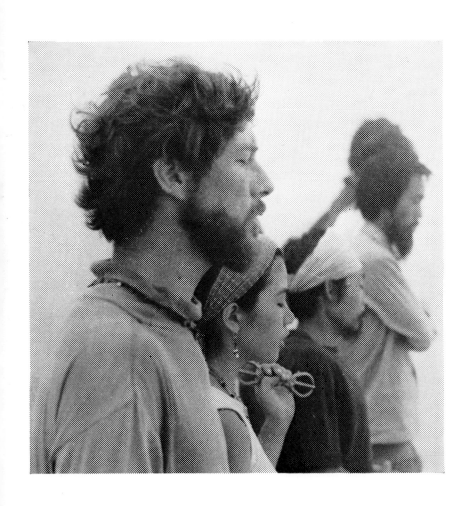

Gary Snyder

six sections from
Mountains
and
Rivers
without end

Fulcrum Press London

Acknowledgements

Parts of this sequence have appeared previously in Origin, Fuck You, A Magazine of the Arts, City Lights Journal, the Doubleday Anchor anthology *A Controversy of Poets* and the Penguin anthology *The New Writing in the U.S.A.* Particular acknowledgement to Donald Allen of Four Seasons Foundation in which these appeared as Writing 9 of the series.
Typography by Stuart Montgomery. The photograph on the cover is by Banyan Ashram. All rights reserved. No part of this book may be reproduced without the written permission of the publisher. Of this first edition one hundred copies are printed on sage glastonbury and are numbered and signed by the author.

Other books by Gary Snyder

Riprap
Myths & Texts
Riprap & Cold Mountain Poems
A Range of Poems (*Collected Poems* Fulcrum Press 1966)
The Back Country (Fulcrum Press 1967)

The Six Sections

from mountains and rivers without end

Bubbs Creek Haircut

for Locke McCorkle

section one

High ceilingd and the double mirrors, the
        calendar a splendid alpine scene — scab barber —
in stained white barber gown, alone, sat down, old man
A summer fog gray San Francisco day
I walked right in. on Howard street
                haircut a dollar twenty-five.
Just clip it close as it will go.
        "now why you want your hair cut back like that."
    —well I : m going to the Sierras for a while
Bubbs Creek and on across to upper Kern.
                he wriggled clippers,
"Well I been up there, I built the cabin
    up at Cedar Grove. In nineteen five."
                old haircut smell

Next door, Goodwill.
                where I came out.
A search for sweater, and a stroll
                in the board & concrete room of
        unfixed junk downstair —
All emblems of the past — too close —
    heaped up in chilly dust and bare bulb glare
Of tables, wheelchairs, battered trunks & wheels
& pots that boiled up coffee nineteen ten, *things*
Swimming on their own & finally freed
                from human need. Or?
        waiting a final flicker of desire

9

To tote them out once more. Some freakish use.
The Master of the limbo drag-leggd watches
                              making prices
        to the people seldom buy
The sag-asst rocker has to make it now. Alone.

                    A few weeks later drove with Locke
    down San Joaquin, us barefoot in the heat
    stopping for beer & melon on the way
                    the Giant Orange,
    rubber shreds of cast truck retreads on the pebble
    shoulders, highway ninety-nine.
                        Sierras marked by cumulus
                        in the east.
        car coughing in the groves,   six thousand feet;
        down to Kings River Canyon; camped at Cedar Grove.
                    hard granite canyon walls that
                    leave no scree

Once tried a haircut at the Barber College too —
Sat half an hour before they told me
                white men use the other side.
Goodwill, St. Vincent de Paul,
                Salvation Army, up the coast
For mackinaws and boots and heavy socks
        —Seattle has the best for logger gear
Once found a pair of good tricouni
        at the under-the-public-market store,
        Mark Tobey's scene,
                torn down I hear —
& Filson jacket with a birdblood stain.

A. G. & me got winter clothes for almost nothing
        at Lake Union, telling the old gal
        we was on our way
To work the winter out up in B. C.
                        hitch-hiking home the
Green hat got a ride (of that more later)

hiking up Bubbs creek saw the trail crew tent
in a scraggly grove of creekside lodgepole pine
                    talked to the guy, he says
"If you see McCool on the other trailcrew over there
tell him Moorehead says to go to hell."
late snow that summer. Crossing the scarred bare
                    shed of Forester Pass
        the winding rock-braced switchbacks
dive in snowbanks, we climb on where
                    pack trains have to dig or wait.
a half iced-over lake, twelve thousand feet
                    its sterile boulder bank
but filled with leaping trout:
                    reflections wobble in the
mingling circles always spreading out
        the crazy web of wavelets makes sense
        seen from high above.
the realm of fallen rock.
a deva world of sorts — it's high
            it is a view that few men see, a point
        bare sunlight
        on the spaces
empty sky
            moulding to fit the shape of what ice left
of fire-thrust, or of tilted, twisted, faulted
            cast-out from this lava belly globe.

The boulder in my minds eye is a chair.
                . . . why was the man drag legg'd?
King of Hell
            or is it a paradise of sorts, thus freed
From acting out the function some
                    creator/carpenter
Thrust on a thing to think he made, himself,
        an object always "chair"
                    Sinister ritual histories.
        is the Mountain God a gimp?
"le Roi Boeuf" and the ritual limp?
                        Good   Will?

Daughter of mountains, stoopt
        moon breast Parvati
  mountain thunder speaks
  hair tingling static as the lightning lashes
  is neither word of love or wisdom;
  though this be danger: hence thee fear.
        Some flowing girl
  whose slippery dance
  untrances Shiva
           —the valley spirit/ Anahita,
              Sarasvati,
  dark and female gate of all the world
  water that cuts backs quartzflake sand
        Soft is the dance that melts the
  mat-haired mountain sitter
      to leap in fire
  & make of sand a tree
      of tree a board, of board (ideas!)
      somebody's rocking chair.
  a room of empty sun of peaks and ridges
      beautiful spirits,
           rocking lotus throne:
  a universe of junk, all left alone.

The hat I always take on mountains:
When we came back down through Oregon
        (three years before)
At nightfall in the Siskiyou few cars pass
A big truck stopped a hundred yards above
    "Siskiyou Stoneware" on the side
The driver said
He recognized my old green hat.
I'd had a ride
    with him two years before
A whole state north
    when hitching down to Portland
        from Warm Springs.

Allen in the rear on straw
   forgot salami   and we went on south
   all night — in many cars — to Berkeley in the dawn.

     upper Kern River country now after nine days walk
     it finally rain.
         we ran on that other trail crew
     setting up new camp in the drizzly pine
     cussing & slapping bugs, 4 days from road,
     we saw McCool, & he said tell that Moorehead
            KISS MY ASS
     we squatted smoking by the fire.
         "I'll never get a green hat now"
     the foreman says   fifty mosquitoes sitting on the brim
                          they must like green.
     & two more days of thundershower and cold
            (on Whitney hair on end
            hail stinging barelegs in the blast of wind
            but yodel off the summit echoes clean)

         all this came after:
Purity of the mountains and goodwills.
The diamond drill of racing icemelt waters
         and bumming trucks & watching
Buildings raze
       the garbage acres burning at the Bay
       the girl who was the skid-row
Cripple's daughter —

          out of the memory of smoking pine
The lotion and the spittoon glitter rises
Chair turns and in the double mirror waver
The old man cranks me down and cracks a chuckle

        "your Bubbs Creek haircut, boy."

                            20. IV. 60

The Elwha River

section two

1

I was a girl waiting by the roadside for my boyfriend to come in
his car. I was pregnant, I should have been going to high school.
I walked up the road when he didn't come, over a bridge; I saw
a sleeping man. I came to the Elwha River — grade school —
classes — I went and sat down with the children. The teacher was
young and sad-looking, homely; she assigned us an essay:
"What I Just Did."

"I was waiting for my boyfriend by the Elwha bridge. The bridge
was redwood, a fresh bridge with inner bark still clinging on some
logs — it smelled good. There was a man there sleeping under redwood trees. He had a box of flies by his head; he was on the ground.
I crossed the Elwha River by a meadow; it had a flat stony prong
between two river forks . . ."

Thinking this would please the teacher. We handed all the papers
in, and got them back — mine was C minus. The children then
went home; the teacher came to me and said "I don't like you."
"Why?"
— "Because I used to be a whore."

The Elwha River, I explained, is a real river, but not the river I
described. Where I had just walked was real but for the dream
river — actually the Elwha doesn't fork at that point.

15

As I write this I must remind myself that there is another Elwha, the actual Olympic peninsula river, which is not the river I took pains to recollect as real in the dream.

There are no redwoods north of southern
Curry County, Oregon.

21. X. 1958

2

Marble hollow-ground hunting knife;

       pigleather tobacco pouch
       left on the ground at Whiskey Bend along
       the Elwha, 1950 —

Sewing kit. Blown off the cot beside me
on the boatdeck by a sudden wind
                   South China Sea;

A black beret Joanne had given me for my birthday
left in some
Kawaramachi bar.

Swiss army knife stole from my pants
       at Juhu Beach outside Bombay,
             a fine italic pen,

Theodora, Kitty-chan,
       bottle of wine got broke.
       things left on the sand.

Lost things.

3

Elwha, from its source. Threadwhite falls
out of snow-tunnel mouths with
cold mist-breath
saddles of deep snow on the ridges —

    o wise stream — o living flow
  o milky confluence, bank cutter
      alder toppler
      make meander,
swampy acres   elk churned mud

The big Douglas fir in this valley.
Nobly groovd bark, it adapts :   where Sitka spruce
cannot.
      Redwood and sequoia
resisting and enduring, as against adaptation;
one mind.

Trail crew foreman says they finally got wise
to making trails low on the outside, so water
can run off good — before they were worried because
packstock always walks the outside of the trail
because they don't want to bump their loads on rocks
or trees. "punching out all the way from N Fork
over Low Divide & clear back here, this punchin gets
mighty old"

Puncheon slab saw cut *wowed*

"They got rip-cut chains now maybe different rakers
this here punchin gets old"

About 12:30 come to Whiskey Bend.
That lowland smell.

21. VIII. 1964

17

Night Highway Ninety-Nine

. . . only the very poor, or eccentric, can surround themselves with shapes of elegance (soon to be demolished) in which they are forced by poverty to move with leisurely grace. We remain alert so as not to get run down, but it turns out you only have to hop a few feet, to one side, and the whole huge machinery rolls by, not seeing you at all.

— Lew Welch

section three

1

We're on our way
        man
      out of town
     go hitching down
   that highway ninety-nine

Too cold and rainy to go out on the Sound
Sitting in Ferndale drinking coffee
Baxter in black, been to a funeral
Raymond in Bellingham — Helena Hotel —
Can't go to Mexico with that weak heart
Well you boys can go south. I stay here.
Fix up a shack — get a part-time job —
        (he disappeared later
         maybe found in the river)
In Ferndale & Bellingham
Went out on trailcrews
Glacier and Marblemount
There we part.

             tiny men with moustaches
             driving ox-teams
             deep in the cedar groves.
             wet brush, tin pants, snoose

Split-shake roof barns
        over berryfields
                white birch chickencoop

Put up in Dick Meigs cabin
                out behind the house —
Coffeecan, PA tin, rags, dirty cups,
Kindling fell behind the stove
                            miceshit
            old magazines,

                    winter's coming in the mountains
                    shut down the show
                    the punks go back to school
                    & the rest hit the road

        strawberries picked, shakeblanks split
        fires all out and the packstrings brought
        down to the valleys
                    set to graze

Gray wharves and hacksaw gothic homes
Shingle mills and stump farms
                            overgrown.

2

Fifty drunk Indians   *Mt. Vernon*
Sleep in the bus station
Strawberry pickers speaking Kwakiutl
            turn at Burlington for Skagit
                        & Ross Dam

        under appletrees by the river
        banks of junkd cars

            B. C. drivers give hitch-hikers rides

"The sheriff's posse stood in double rows   *Everett*
        flogged the naked Wobblies down
        with stalks of Devil's Club
        & run them out of town"

While shingle-weavers lost their fingers
        in the tricky feed and take
        of double saws.

Dried, shrimp   *Seattle*
            smoked,   salmon
        — before the war old indian came
& sold us hard-smoked Chinook
From his truck-bed model T
                    Lake City,

        waste of trees & topsoil, beast, herb,
        edible roots, Indian field-farms & white men
        dances   washed, leached, burnt out
        Minds blunt, ug! talk twisted

        A night of the long poem
        and the mined guitar . . .
        "Forming the new society
        within the shell of the old"
            mess of tincan camps and littered roads

The Highway passes straight through
                        every town
At Matsons washing blujeans
            hills and saltwater
                ack, the woodsmoke in my brain

High Olympics — can't go there again

        East Marginal Way the hitch-hike zone
        Boeing down across Duwamish slough

& angle out
        & on.

Night rain wet concrete headlights
               blind   *Tacoma*

      Salt air/   Bulk cargo/   Steam cycle

           AIR REDUCTION

        eating peanuts I don't give a damn
        if anybody ever stops   I'll walk
        to San Francisco   what the hell

               "that's where your going?
               "why you got that pack?

Well man I just don't feel right
Without something on my back

        & this character in milkman overalls
        "I have to come out here
        every onct in a while, there's a guy
        blows me here"

             way out of town.

Stayed in Olympia with Dick Meigs
  — this was a different year & he had moved —
  sleep on a cot in the back yard
  half the night watch falling stars
These guys got babies now
         drink beer, come back from wars
    "I'd like to save up all my money
    get a big new car, go down to Reno
    & latch onto one of those rich girls —
    I'd fix their little ass" — nineteen yr old
    N. Dakota boy fixing to get married next month

22

To Centralia in a purple ford.

                carstruck dead doe
                by the Skookumchuck river

Fat man in a Chevrolet
                wants to go back to L. A.
                "too damnd poor now"
Airbrakes on the log trucks hiss and whine
Stand in the dark by the stoplight.
            big fat cars tool by

Drink coffee, drink more coffee
                    brush teeth back of Shell
        hot shoes
                stay on the rightside of that
                        yellow line

Marys Corner, turn for Mt. Rainier
        — once caught a ride at night for Portland here
Five Mexicans, ask me "chip in on the gas"
        I never was more broke & down.
        got fired that day by the USA
        (the District Ranger up at Packwood
        thought the wobblies had been dead for
                            forty years
        but the FBI smelled treason
                    — my red beard)

That Waco Texas boy
        took A. G. & me through miles of snow
        had a chest of logger gear
        at the home of an Indian girl
        in Kelso, hadn't seen since Fifty-four

Toledo, Castle Rock, free way
            four lane
        no stoplights & no crossings, only cars

& people walking, old hitch-hikers
break the law. How do I know.
                the state cop
                    told me so.

Come a dozen times into
                    Portland
        on the bum or
                    hasty lover
            late   at   night

3

Portland

dust kicking up behind the trucks — night rides —
who waits in the coffee stop
                    night highway 99

        Sokei-an met an old man on the banks of the
        Columbia river growing potatoes & living all alone,
        Sokei-an asked him the reason why he lived there,
        he said
        Boy, no one ever asked me the reason why.
        I like to be alone.
        I am an old man.
        I have forgotten how to speak human words.

All night freezing
        in the back of a truck
    dawn at Smith river
        battering on in loggers pickups
                    prunes for lunch
The next night, Siuslaw.

Portland sawdust   down town
Buttermilk corner,   all you want for a nickel
    (now a dime)

                    — Sujata gave Gautama
                                    buttermilk,
            (No doubt! says Sokei-an, that's all it was
                            plain buttermilk.)

            rim of mountains.   pulp bark chewd snag
                                    papermill
            tugboom in the river
            — used to lean on bridgerails
            dreaming up eruptions and quakes —

Slept under Juniper in the Siskiyou   (Yreka)
        a sleeping bag, a foot of snow
        black rolled umbrella
        ice slick asphalt

Caught a ride the only car come by
        at seven in the morning
        chewing froze salami
Riding with a passed-out LA whore
        glove compartment full of booze,
        the driver a rider, nobody cowboy,
        sometime hood,
Like me picked up to drive,
        & drive the blues away.
                we drank to Portland
                        & we treated that girl good.

I split my last two bucks with him in town
        went out to Carol & Billy's in the woods.

    — foggy morning in Newport
        housetrailers
                under the fir.

An old book on Japan at the Goodwill
        unfurld umbrella in the sailing snow
                sat back in black wood

                    barber college
                  chair, a shave
On Second Street in Portland
                  what elegance.   What a life.

          bust my belly with a quart of
                              buttermilk
          & five dry heels of French bread
          from the market cheap
                    clean shaved, dry feet,

We're on our way
                  man
                        out of town
Go hitching down that
                  highway ninety-nine.

4

Oil-pump broken, motor burning out   *Salem*

Ex-logger selling skidder cable
     wants to get to San Francisco,
     fed and drunk   *Eugene*

Guy just back from Alaska — don't like
     the States, there's too much law   *Sutherlin*

A woman with a kid & two bales of hay.   *Roseburg*

Sawmill worker, young guy thinking of
     going to Eureka for redwood logging
     later in the year   *Dillard*

Two Assembly of God Pentecostal boys in
     a Holy Roller High School. One had
                  spoken in
                        tongues.   *Canyonville*

26

LASME   Los-Angeles—Seattle Motor Express

place on highway 20:   LITTLE ELK
                        badger & badger

South of Yoncalla burn the engine
                    run out of oil

Yaquina fishdocks
                candlefish & perch
                slant-faced woman fishing
            tuna stacked like cordwood
            the once-glimpsed-into door
                        company freezer shed
            a sick old seagull settles
            down to die.
            the ordinary, casual, ruffle of the
                        tail & wings.
(Six great highways; so far only one)

            freshwater creeks on the beach sand
                at Kalaloch I caught a bag of water
            at Agate Beach
                made a diversion with my toe

Jumpoff Joe Creek &
            a man carrying nothing, walking sort of
            stiff-legged along, blue jeans & denim jacket,
            wrinkled face, just north of
            Louse Creek

                — Abandon really means it
                — the network womb stretched loose all
                                    things slip
                        through

Dreaming on a bench under newspapers
I woke covered over with Rhododendron blooms
Alone in a State Park in Oregon.

"I had a girl in Oakland who worked
for a doctor, she was a nurse, she let him
eat her. She died of tuberculosis   *Grants*
& I drove back that night   *Pass*
                    to Portland
non stop, crying all the way."

        "I picked up a young mother with two
        children once, their house had just
                        burned down"
        "I picked up an Italian tree-surgeon
        in Port Angeles once, he had all his
        saws and tools all screwed & bolted on
                a beat up bike"

Oxyoke, Wolf Creek,

A guy coming off a five-day binge, to   *Phoenix*

An ex-bartender from Lebanon, to   *Redding*

Man & wife on a drinking spree, to   *Anderson*

Snow on the pines & firs around Lake Shasta
        — Chinese scene of winter hills & trees
            us "little travellers" in the bitter cold

                six-lane highway slash & DC twelves
                bridge building   squat earth-movers
        — yellow bugs

            I speak for hawks.

The road that's followed goes forever;
In half a minute crossed and left behind.

Out of the snow and into red-dirt plains

blossoming plums

Each time you go that road it gets more straight
curves across the mountains lost in fill
towns you had to slow down all four lane
Azalea, Myrtle Creek
WATCH OUT FOR DEER

At Project City Indian hitcher
Standing under single tarpole lamp
nobody stopped
Ginsberg & I walked
four miles & camped by an oak fire
left by the road crew

Going to San Francisco
Yeah San Francisco
Yeah we came from Seattle
Even farther north
Yeah we been working in the mountains
in the Spring
in the Autumn
always go this highway ninety-nine —

"I was working in a mill three weeks there
then it burned down & the guy didn't even
pay us off — but I can do anything —
I'll go to San Francisco — tend bar"

Standing in the night.
In the world-end winds
By the overpass bridge

Junction US 40 and Highway Ninety-nine

Trucks, trucks,   roll by
Kicking up dust — dead flowers —

Sixteen speeds forward
Windows open
Stoppd at the edge of Willows for a bite

                    grass shoots on the edge of
                    drained rice plains

                              — cheap olives —
Where are the Sierras.

                    level, dry,
Highway turns west

                    miles gone, speed
                                        still
                    pass through lower hills
                    heat dying
                    toward Vallejo
           gray on the salt baywater
              brown grass ridges
                    blue mesquite

One leggd Heron in the tideflats

                    State of Cars.

Sailor getting back to ship
                    — I'm sick of car exhaust

                    City
           gleaming far away

we make it into town tonight
get clean & drink some wine —

SAN FRANCISCO

NO
body
gives a shit
man
who you are or
whats your car
there IS no
ninety-nine.

Hymn To The Goddess
San Francisco
In Paradise

If you want to live high get high
— Nihil C.

section four

1

up under the bell skirt
caving over the soil
white legs flashing
   — amazed to see under their clothes they are
           naked
    this makes them sacred
& more than they are in their own shape
          free.
the wildest cock-blowing
  gang-fucking foul-tongued
      head chick
  thus the most so —

2

high town
high   in the dark   town
      dream   sex   church
      YAHWEH   peyote spook
      Mary the fish-eyed
          spotless,
          lascivious,
vomiting molten gold.

san fran sisco
hung over & swing down

                    dancers on water
            oil slick glide
            shaman longshoremen
            magical strikes —
howls of the guardians rise from the waterfront.
— state line beauties those switcher engines
            leading waggons
warehouz of jewels and fresh fur
car leans
        on its downhill springs
                    parked on mountainsides.
white minarets in the night
    demon fog chaos.
bison stroll on the grass.
    languid and elegant, fucking while standing
                    young couples in silk
                    make-up on.

crystal towers   gleam for a hundred miles
            poison oak hedges, walld child garden
& the ring mountains holding a cool
            basin of pure evening fog
            strained thru the bridge
            gold and orange,
beams of cars wiser than drivers
    stream across promenades, causeways
            incensed exhaust.

smiling the City Hall Altar to Heaven
    they serve up the cock   tail,
there is higher than nature in city
        it spins in the sky.

3

quenching the blue flame
tasting the tea brought from China
cracking the fresh duck egg on white plate

passed out the gates of our chambers
over the clear miles, ships.
forever such ecstasy
        wealth & such beauty
        we live in the sign of Good Will . . .
(the white-robed saint trim my locks for
        a paltry sum . . . life is
        like free)
rolling lawns clippt and the smell of gum tree.
boiled crab from a saltwater vat.
                        rhine wine.
bison and elk of Chrysopylae
eels in those rocks in the wave
olive oil, garlic, soy, hard cheese.

Devas of small merit in Jambudvipa
Plucking sour berries to eat:
shall ascend to an eminence,
scanning the scene
        fog in
    from the Farallones
long ship low   far below
    sliding under the bridge
    bright white.   red-lead.
            — blue of the sea.
    on that ship is me.

4

— smilers all on the nod nap on cots
but the slither   & breakfree
        tossd slipper up on the toe
            & the white thighs open
                the flesh of the wet flower
                    LAW
crossed eyes gleam   *come*
        flowery prints and
            yellow kettles in a row

        breast weight swelld down

kind chairmen smile around,
generals and presidents swallow
                hoping   they too   can come . . . .
        THERE IS NO WAY

        turn back dead tourist
        drop your crumb your funny passport
— fall back richer spenders
        think you make with wild teenager
                on hard forever
                crust in jewel

                — *you are too old.*
the san francisco fake front strip tease
phony, sweaty,
last a minute and they stink and die

THIS LAND IS FOR THE HIGH
        & love is for ten thousand years.
                (damnd square climbers give me pains)
them wilty blossoms on her sweaty brow —
        the flute and lute and drums

        policecars sireen down on Fillmore
        fog clears back away
        the police close in
                & shoot the loose
        & clouds are slipping by

& hide it in your pockets.

It all becomes plain sky.

The Market

section five

1

heart of the city
       down town.
the country   side

John Muir.   up before dawn
packing pears in the best boxes
     beat out the others — to Market
       the Crystal Palace
on the morning milk-run train.

me, milk bottles by bike
guernsey milk, six percent butterfat
raw and left to rise natural
            ten cents a quart
slipped on the frost turning
       in to a driveway
   and broke all nine bottles.
when we had cows.
     a feathery hemlock out back
     by manure pile where
          one cow once
     lay with milkfever   transfusions
     & worries until the vet come
we do this still dark in the morning —

to town on high thin-wheeled carts.
squat on the boxtop stall.
papayas   banana   sliced fish   grated ginger

fruit for fish, meat for flowers
        french bread for ladle
              steamer, tea giant
        rough glaze earthware
                  — for brass shrine bowls.

push through fish
bound pullets lay on their sides
                        wet slab
watch us with glimmering eye
                        slosh water.
a carrot, a lettuce.   a ball of cookd noodle.
        beggars hang by the flower stall
        give them all some

strong women.   dirt from the hills
                        in her nails.

valley thatch houses
      palmgroves for hedges
ricefield and thrasher
        to white rice
        dongs and piastre
to market, the
              changes, how much
              is our change:

2

seventy-five feet hoed rows equals
one hour explaining power steering
equals two big crayfish =
         all the buttermilk you can drink
= twelve pounds cauliflower
= five cartons greek olives = hitch-hiking
         from Ogden Utah to Burns Oregon
= aspirin, iodine, and bandages
= a lay in Naples = beef
= lamb ribs   = Patna
                    long grain rice, eight pounds
equals two kilogram soybeans = a boxwood
                         geisha comb.
equals the whole family at the movies
equals whipping dirty clothes on rocks
  three days, some Indian river
= piecing off beggars two weeks
= bootlace and shoelace
      equals one gross inflatable
      plastic pillows
= a large box of petit-fours, chou-crêmes —
      barley-threshing
 • mangoes, apples, custard apples, raspberries
= picking three flats strawberries
= a christmas tree = a taxi ride
carrots, daikon, eggplant, greenpeppers,
oregano   white   goat   cheese
      = a fresh-eyed bonito, live clams.
a swordfish
a salmon
  a handful of silvery smelt in the pocket;
      whiskey in cars.   out late after dates.
      old folks   eating cake   in secret
      breastmilk enough.
                if the belly be fed —

& wash-down.   hose off aisles
reach under fruitstands
     green gross rack
        meat scum on chop blocks
        bloody butcher concrete floor
      old knives sharpened down to scalpels
        brown wrap paper rolls, stiff
          push-broom back
wet spilld food
      when the market is closed
        the cleanup comes
         equals

a billygoat pushing through people
stinking and grabbing a cabbage
arrogant, tough,
he took it — they let him —
Katmandu — the market

I gave a man seventy paise
in return for a clay pot
of curds
was it worth it?
how can I tell

3

they eat feces
    in the dark
    on stone floors.
one legged animals, hopping cows
    limping dogs   blind cats

crunching garbage in the market
    broken fingers
        cabbage
    head on the ground.

who has young face.
             open pit eyes
between the bullock carts and people
    head pivot with the footsteps
                              passing by
dark scrotum spilld on the street
       penis laid by his thigh
                    torso
turns with the sun

I came to buy
       a few bananas by the ganges
          while waiting for my wife.

Journeys

section six

1

Genji caught a gray bird, fluttering. It
was wounded, so I hit it with a coal shovel.
It stiffened, grew straight and symmetrical,
and began to increase in size. I took it by
the head with both hands and held it as it
swelled, turning the head from side to side.
It turned into a woman, and I was embracing
her. We walked down a dim-lighted stairway
holding hands, walking more and more swiftly
through an enormous maze, all underground.
Occasionally we touched surface, and redescended.
As we walked I kept a chart of our route in
mind — but it became increasingly complex — and
just when we reached the point where I was
about to lose my grasp of it, the woman trans-
ferred a piece of fresh-tasting apple from her
mouth to mine. Then I woke.

2

Through deep forests to the coast,
and stood on a white sandspit looking in :
over lowland swamps and prairies
where no man had ever been
to a chill view of the Olympics, in a chill clear wind.

3

We moved across dark stony ground to the great
wall: hundreds of feet high. What was beyond
it, cows? — then a thing began to rise
up from behind.
I shot my arrows, shot arrows at it, but it came —
until we turned and ran, "It's too big to
fight" — the rising thing a quarter mile across —
it was the flaming, pulsing sun. We fled and
stumbled on the bright lit plain.

4

Where were we —
A girl in a red skirt, high heels,
going up the stairs before me in a made-over barn.
White-wash peeling, we lived together in the loft,
on cool bare boards.
— lemme tell you something kid —
        back in 1910.

5

Walking a dusty road through plowed-up fields
at forest-fire time — the fir tree hills dry,
smoke of the far fires blurred the air —
& passed on into woods, along a pond,
beneath a big red cedar,
to a bank of blinding blue wild flowers
and thick green grass on levelled ground
of hillside where our old house used to stand.
I saw the footings damp and tangled,
and thought my father was in jail,
and wondered why my mother never died,
and thought I ought to bring my sister back.

6

High up in a yellow-gold
dry range of mountains —
brushy, rocky, cactussy hills
slowly hiking down — finally can see below,
a sea of clouds.

Lower down, always moving slowly over the
dry ground descending, can see through breaks
in the clouds: flat land.
Damp green level ricefields, farm houses,
at last to feel the heat and damp.

Descending to this humid, clouded, level world:
now I have come to the LOWLANDS.

7

Underground building chambers clogged with refuse heaps
discarded furniture, slag, old nails,
rotting plaster, faint wisps — antique newspapers
rattle in the winds that come forever down the hall.
ladders
passing, climbing, and stopping, on from door to door.
one tiny light bulb left still burning
             — now the last —
locked *inside* is hell.
Movies going, men milling round the posters
          in shreds
          the movie always running
— we all head in here somewhere;

— years just looking for the bathrooms.
Huge and filthy, with strange-shaped toilets full of shit.
Dried shit all around, smeared across the walls of the
adjoining room,
and a vast hat rack.

8

With Lew rode in a bus over the mountains —
rutted roads along the coast of Washington
through groves of redwoods. Sitting in the
back of an almost-empty bus,
talking and riding through.
Yellow leaves fluttering down. Passing
through tiny towns at times. Damp cabins
set in dark groves of trees.
Beaches with estuaries and sandbars. I brought
a woman here once long ago,
but passed on through too quick.

9

We were following a long river into the mountains.
Finally we rounded a ridge and could see deeper in —
the farther peaks stony and barren, a few alpine
trees.
Ko-san and I stood on a point by a cliff, over a
rock-walled canyon. Ko said, "Now we have come to
where we die." I asked him, what's that up there,
then — meaning the further mountains.
"That's the world after death." I thought it looked
just like the land we'd been travelling, and couldn't
see why we should have to die.
Ko grabbed me and pulled me over the cliff —
both of us falling. I hit and I was dead. I saw
my body for a while, then it was gone. Ko was
there too. We were at the bottom of the gorge.
We started drifting up the canyon, "This is the
way to the back country."